NATURAL HOME REMEDY FOR CHOLESTEROL MANAGEMENT

Gideon Oow

Table of Contents

Introduction

- Other Contributing Factors (Age, Gender, etc.)

Chapter 3: Symptoms of High Cholesterol

- Recognizing the Signs
- How High Cholesterol is Diagnosed
- The Silent Nature of High Cholesterol

Chapter 4: The Dangers of High Cholesterol

- Cardiovascular Disease
- Stroke
- Peripheral Artery Disease
- Other Health Risks

Chapter 5: Benefits of Natural Remedies

- Why Choose Natural Remedies?
- The Science Behind Natural Ingredients

Chapter 11: Lemon for Cholesterol Control

- Nutritional Benefits of Lemon
- Lemon's Role in Cholesterol Management
- Recipes and Usage Tips for Lemon
- Precautions and Considerations

Chapter 12: Natural Remedy for Cholesterol Management

Introduction

In today's fast-paced world, the prevalence of high cholesterol levels has become a significant health concern. High cholesterol, if left unchecked, can lead to serious health complications such as cardiovascular disease, stroke, and peripheral artery disease. While medication is often prescribed to manage cholesterol levels, there is a growing interest in natural remedies that can help lower cholesterol without the side effects of pharmaceuticals.

This book explores the power of natural remedies in managing cholesterol, focusing on ingredients that are readily available and easy to incorporate into daily life. The remedies discussed include garlic, onion, turmeric, lime, lemon, and clove, each offering unique benefits for cholesterol management. By understanding the science behind these natural ingredients and learning how to use them effectively, readers can take proactive steps towards improving their cholesterol levels and overall health.

The Purpose of This Book

The primary purpose of this book is to provide readers with comprehensive information about cholesterol, its causes, symptoms, and dangers, while offering practical guidance on how to manage and lower cholesterol levels naturally. By highlighting the benefits of natural remedies and providing detailed instructions on their usage, this book aims to empower readers to take control of their health and well-being.

What to Expect

In the following chapters, we will delve into the world of cholesterol, exploring its impact on health and the body. We will discuss the various causes of high cholesterol, the symptoms to watch out for, and the potential dangers of untreated high cholesterol. We will also explore the benefits of natural remedies, focusing on garlic, onion, turmeric, lime, lemon, and clove, and how they can be used to lower cholesterol levels effectively.

Each chapter will provide detailed information on the nutritional and medicinal properties of these natural ingredients, as well as practical tips on how to incorporate them into your daily routine. We will also discuss complementary lifestyle changes that can help improve cholesterol levels, such as diet, exercise, stress management, and avoiding harmful habits.

How to Use This Book

This book is designed to be a practical guide for anyone looking to manage their cholesterol levels naturally. Whether you are already dealing with high cholesterol or are looking to prevent it, the information and tips provided in this book can help you make informed decisions about your health. Each chapter is structured to provide you with the knowledge and tools you need to take action towards better cholesterol management.

We encourage you to read through the chapters at your own pace, taking notes and reflecting on how you can apply the information to your own life. The recipes and usage tips provided are meant to be simple and accessible, allowing you to easily incorporate these natural remedies into your daily routine. Remember, small changes can lead to significant improvements in your cholesterol levels and overall health.

The Journey Ahead

As you embark on this journey towards better cholesterol management, we hope that this book will serve as a valuable resource and guide. By embracing natural remedies and making positive lifestyle changes, you can take control of your cholesterol levels and improve your overall health and well-being. Let's begin this journey together, towards a healthier, happier you.

Chapter 1

Understanding Cholesterol

Cholesterol is a waxy, fat-like substance that is found in the cells of your body and in your blood. While cholesterol is essential for building healthy cells and producing hormones, too much cholesterol in the blood can lead to health problems. In this chapter, we will explore what cholesterol is, the different types of cholesterol, and its role in the body.

What is Cholesterol?

Cholesterol is a lipid, a type of fat that is produced by the liver and is also found in certain foods. It is an essential component of cell membranes and is used by the body to produce hormones, vitamin D, and bile acids that help digest fats. Cholesterol is transported in the blood by lipoproteins, which are particles made up of fat and protein.

Types of Cholesterol: LDL, HDL, and Triglycerides

There are several types of cholesterol, but the two most commonly known are low-density lipoprotein (LDL) cholesterol and high-density lipoprotein (HDL) cholesterol.

- LDL Cholesterol: LDL cholesterol is often referred to as "bad" cholesterol because high levels can lead to the buildup of plaque in the arteries, which can increase the risk of heart disease and stroke.
- HDL Cholesterol: HDL cholesterol is known as "good" cholesterol because it helps remove LDL cholesterol from the arteries, reducing the risk of heart disease.
- Triglycerides: Triglycerides are another type of fat found in the blood. High levels of triglycerides, like high levels of LDL cholesterol, can increase the risk of heart disease.

The Role of Cholesterol in the Body

Cholesterol plays a vital role in the body's normal functioning, but too much cholesterol can be harmful. When there is an excess of cholesterol in the blood, it can build up in the walls of the arteries, forming plaque. Over time, this plaque can narrow the arteries, reducing blood flow and increasing the risk of heart attack and stroke.

Cholesterol levels can be influenced by a variety of factors, including diet, weight, physical activity, age, and genetics. While some risk factors, such as age and genetics, cannot be changed, others, such as diet and exercise, can be modified to help manage cholesterol levels.

Understanding cholesterol and its role in the body is the first step towards managing and lowering cholesterol levels. In the following chapters, we will explore natural remedies and lifestyle changes that

can help you take control of your cholesterol levels

and improve your overall health.

Chapter 2

Causes of High Cholesterol

High cholesterol, also known as hypercholesterolemia, is a common condition that can increase the risk of heart disease and stroke. In this chapter, we will explore the various causes of high cholesterol, including dietary factors, genetic predisposition, lifestyle choices, and other contributing factors.

Dietary Factors

Diet plays a significant role in cholesterol levels. Foods that are high in saturated and trans fats can raise LDL cholesterol levels, increasing the risk of heart disease. Examples of foods high in these unhealthy fats include:

- Fried foods
- Processed foods

- Fatty cuts of meat
- Full-fat dairy products
- Baked goods made with hydrogenated oils

On the other hand, foods high in fiber, such as fruits, vegetables, whole grains, and legumes, can help lower cholesterol levels by reducing the absorption of cholesterol in the intestines.

Genetic Predisposition

Genetics can also play a role in cholesterol levels. Some people inherit genes that cause their bodies to produce too much cholesterol. This condition, known as familial hypercholesterolemia, can lead to very high cholesterol levels from a young age and increase the risk of early heart disease.

Lifestyle Factors

Lifestyle choices can significantly impact cholesterol levels. Lack of physical activity can lower HDL cholesterol levels and lead to weight gain, both of which can increase the risk of high cholesterol. Smoking can also lower HDL cholesterol levels and damage the walls of the arteries, making it easier for plaque to build up.

Other Contributing Factors

Other factors that can contribute to high cholesterol include:

- Age: Cholesterol levels tend to rise with age.
- Gender: Before menopause, women typically have lower total cholesterol levels than men of the same age. After menopause, however, women's LDL cholesterol levels often increase.
- Weight: Excess weight can lead to higher LDL cholesterol levels and lower HDL cholesterol levels.
- Medical Conditions: Certain medical conditions, such as diabetes, hypothyroidism, and kidney disease, can affect cholesterol levels.

High cholesterol is a common condition that can have serious health consequences if left untreated. By understanding the various causes of high cholesterol, you can take steps to manage and lower your cholesterol levels. In the following chapters, we will explore natural remedies and lifestyle changes that can help you improve your cholesterol levels and reduce your risk of heart disease and stroke.

Chapter 3

Symptoms of High Cholesterol

High cholesterol is often referred to as a "silent" condition because it typically does not cause any symptoms until it leads to more serious health problems. In this chapter, we will explore the symptoms of high cholesterol, how it is diagnosed, and the importance of regular cholesterol screenings.

Recognizing the Signs

While high cholesterol itself does not usually cause symptoms, it can lead to conditions that do have noticeable symptoms, such as:

- Chest pain (angina) or chest tightness
- Pain in the legs, arms, or elsewhere due to narrowed arteries (peripheral artery disease)
- Stroke
- Heart attack

- Yellowish deposits of cholesterol around the eyes (xanthomas)

How High Cholesterol is Diagnosed

High cholesterol is typically diagnosed through a blood test called a lipid panel. This test measures the levels of cholesterol and triglycerides in your blood. Your doctor may recommend regular cholesterol screenings based on your age, risk factors, and family history.

The Silent Nature of High Cholesterol

One of the challenges of high cholesterol is its silent nature. Many people with high cholesterol are unaware of their condition until it leads to more serious health problems, such as heart disease or stroke. This is why regular cholesterol screenings are so important, especially if you have risk factors such as a family history of high cholesterol or heart disease, smoking, obesity, or an unhealthy diet.

High cholesterol is often a "silent" condition, meaning it typically does not cause symptoms until it leads to more serious health problems. Recognizing the signs of high cholesterol and understanding the importance of regular cholesterol screenings can help you take proactive steps to manage and lower your cholesterol levels. In the following chapters, we will explore natural remedies and lifestyle changes that can help you improve your cholesterol levels and reduce your risk of heart disease and stroke.

Chapter 4

The Dangers of High Cholesterol

High cholesterol levels can have serious health consequences if left untreated. In this chapter, we will explore the dangers of high cholesterol, including its impact on cardiovascular health, stroke risk, and other health risks.

Cardiovascular Disease

One of the primary dangers of high cholesterol is its association with cardiovascular disease. High levels of LDL cholesterol can lead to the buildup of plaque in the arteries, a condition known as atherosclerosis. Over time, this plaque can narrow the arteries and restrict blood flow to the heart, increasing the risk of heart attack and angina (chest pain).

Stroke

High cholesterol is also a significant risk factor for stroke. If a plaque in the arteries ruptures, it can form a blood clot that can block blood flow to the brain, leading to a stroke. Atherosclerosis in the carotid arteries, which supply blood to the brain, is a common cause of stroke associated with high cholesterol.

Peripheral Artery Disease (PAD)

High cholesterol can also lead to peripheral artery disease (PAD), a condition in which plaque buildup narrows the arteries that supply blood to the limbs, usually the legs. PAD can cause leg pain, numbness, and difficulty walking, and in severe cases, it can lead to gangrene and amputation.

Other Health Risks

In addition to cardiovascular disease, stroke, and PAD, high cholesterol is also associated with other health risks, including:

- High blood pressure
- Diabetes
- Gallstones
- Metabolic syndrome

High cholesterol is not just a number on a lab report—it is a significant risk factor for serious health conditions. Understanding the dangers of high cholesterol and taking steps to manage and lower your cholesterol levels can help reduce your risk of heart disease, stroke, and other health problems. In the following chapters, we will explore natural remedies and lifestyle changes that can help you improve your cholesterol levels and protect your cardiovascular health.

Chapter 5

Benefits of Natural Remedies

Natural remedies offer a holistic approach to managing high cholesterol, providing benefits beyond just lowering cholesterol levels. In this chapter, we will explore the advantages of using natural remedies such as garlic, onion, turmeric, lime, lemon, and clove to improve cholesterol levels and overall health.

Why Choose Natural Remedies?

Natural remedies are often preferred over pharmaceuticals due to their potential for fewer side effects and their ability to address underlying health issues. Natural remedies work with the body's natural processes to promote healing and balance, rather than simply masking symptoms.

The Science Behind Natural Ingredients

Many natural ingredients have been studied for their cholesterol-lowering effects. For example, garlic has been shown to lower total cholesterol and LDL cholesterol levels, while increasing HDL cholesterol levels. Turmeric contains curcumin, a compound with antioxidant and anti-inflammatory properties that may help lower cholesterol levels. Lime and lemon are rich in vitamin C and antioxidants, which can help reduce inflammation and lower cholesterol levels. Clove has been shown to lower LDL cholesterol levels and triglycerides, while increasing HDL cholesterol levels.

Incorporating Natural Remedies Into Your Routine

One of the benefits of natural remedies is their versatility and ease of use. For example, garlic can be added to a wide variety of dishes, while turmeric can be used in curries, soups, and smoothies. Lime and lemon can be used to flavor water, salads, and other dishes, while clove can be added to baked goods and savory dishes.

Supporting Overall Health and Well-being
In addition to their cholesterol-lowering effects, natural remedies offer a range of other health benefits. For example, garlic has antibacterial and antiviral properties, while turmeric has been shown to reduce inflammation and improve digestion. Lime and lemon are rich in vitamin C, which is essential for immune function, while clove has been used for its pain-relieving and antimicrobial properties.

Natural remedies offer a safe and effective way to manage high cholesterol and improve overall health. By incorporating natural ingredients such as garlic, onion, turmeric, lime, lemon, and clove into your diet and lifestyle, you can take proactive steps towards better cholesterol levels and a healthier life. In the following chapters, we will explore each of these natural remedies in more detail, including their nutritional benefits, how they work to lower cholesterol, and practical tips for incorporating them into your daily routine

Chapter 6

Garlic for Managing Cholesterol

Garlic is a popular natural remedy with a long history of medicinal use, including its ability to lower cholesterol levels. In this chapter, we will explore the health benefits of garlic, its impact on cholesterol levels, and practical tips for incorporating garlic into your diet.

Health Benefits of Garlic

Garlic is rich in sulfur compounds, antioxidants, and other bioactive substances that contribute to its health benefits. These compounds have been shown to have anti-inflammatory, antimicrobial, and immune-boosting properties. Garlic is also known for its cardiovascular benefits, including its ability to lower cholesterol and blood pressure, reduce the risk of heart disease, and improve circulation.

How Garlic Helps Lower Cholesterol

Garlic contains compounds such as allicin, which have been shown to lower LDL cholesterol levels and increase HDL cholesterol levels. Allicin works by inhibiting the enzyme HMG-CoA reductase, which is involved in cholesterol synthesis in the liver. By blocking this enzyme, garlic helps reduce the production of cholesterol in the body, leading to lower overall cholesterol levels.

Recipes and Usage Tips for Garlic

- Raw Garlic: Eating raw garlic is one of the most potent ways to reap its benefits. You can mince garlic and add it to salads, dressings, or dips.
- Cooked Garlic: Cooking garlic can mellow its flavor while still retaining some of its health benefits. Add minced garlic to soups, stews, sauces, or stir-fries.
- Garlic Supplements: If you don't enjoy the taste of garlic or find it difficult to incorporate into your diet, garlic

supplements are available in the form of capsules or tablets.

Precautions and Considerations

While garlic is generally safe for most people when consumed in moderate amounts, it can cause side effects such as bad breath, body odor, and digestive issues in some individuals. If you are taking blood-thinning medications or have a bleeding disorder, consult with your healthcare provider before using garlic supplements, as garlic may increase the risk of bleeding.

Garlic is a versatile and potent natural remedy that offers a range of health benefits, including its ability to lower cholesterol levels. By incorporating garlic into your diet and lifestyle, you can take proactive steps towards improving your cholesterol levels and overall cardiovascular health. In the following chapters, we will explore other natural remedies, including onion, turmeric, lime, lemon, and clove, and how they can help you manage and lower your cholesterol levels naturally.

Chapter 7

Onion and Cholesterol Reduction

Onions are not only a flavorful addition to many dishes but also a natural remedy that may help lower cholesterol levels. In this chapter, we will explore the nutritional profile of onions, how they contribute to cholesterol management, and practical tips for incorporating onions into your diet.

Nutritional Profile of Onions

Onions are low in calories but rich in nutrients. They are a good source of vitamin C, vitamin B6, and dietary fiber. Onions also contain sulfur compounds, flavonoids, and antioxidants, which contribute to their health benefits.

How Onions Help Lower Cholesterol

Onions contain sulfur compounds, such as allyl sulfides, which have been shown to lower LDL cholesterol levels and raise HDL cholesterol levels. These compounds work by inhibiting the production of cholesterol in the liver and increasing the breakdown and excretion of cholesterol from the body.

Recipes and Usage Tips for Onions

- Raw Onions: Adding raw onions to salads, sandwiches, or wraps is a simple way to incorporate them into your diet.

- Cooked Onions: Cooking onions can enhance their flavor and make them more digestible. Saute onions with other vegetables, add them to soups or stews, or use them as a base for sauces and gravies.

- Onion Extract: Onion extract supplements are also available and may be beneficial for those who do not enjoy the taste of onions or have difficulty digesting them.

Precautions and Considerations

While onions are generally safe for most people when consumed in moderation, they can cause digestive issues such as gas, bloating, and heartburn in some individuals. If you have a known allergy to onions, avoid consuming them or consult with your healthcare provider before doing so.

Onions are not only a flavorful addition to your meals but also a natural remedy that may help lower cholesterol levels. By incorporating onions into your diet in various ways, you can enjoy their health benefits and take proactive steps towards managing and lowering your cholesterol levels. In the following chapters, we will explore other natural remedies, including turmeric, lime, lemon, garlic, and clove, and how they can help you improve your cholesterol levels and overall health.

Chapter 8

The Power of Turmeric in Cholesterol Management

Turmeric is a vibrant yellow spice commonly used in Indian cuisine and traditional medicine. It contains a compound called curcumin, which is believed to have a range of health benefits, including the potential to lower cholesterol levels. In this chapter, we will explore the nutritional and medicinal properties of turmeric, its role in cholesterol management, and practical tips for incorporating turmeric into your diet.

Nutritional and Medicinal Properties of Turmeric

Turmeric is rich in antioxidants and has anti-inflammatory properties, thanks to its active compound, curcumin. Curcumin has been studied for its potential to reduce inflammation, improve cognitive function, and lower the risk of chronic diseases such as heart disease and cancer.

Turmeric's Role in Cholesterol Management

Studies suggest that curcumin may help lower LDL cholesterol levels and triglycerides, while increasing HDL cholesterol levels. Curcumin is believed to work by reducing the production of cholesterol in the liver and increasing the excretion of cholesterol from the body. It also has antioxidant properties that may protect against the oxidation of LDL cholesterol, which is believed to contribute to the development of atherosclerosis.

Recipes and Usage Tips for Turmeric

- Golden Milk: A popular way to consume turmeric is by making golden milk, a beverage made by simmering turmeric with milk and other spices. This soothing drink is often enjoyed before bedtime.

- Curries and Stews: Turmeric is a key ingredient in many curry powders and is commonly used in curries, stews, and soups to add flavor and color.
- Turmeric Tea: You can also make turmeric tea by steeping turmeric powder or fresh turmeric slices in hot water. Add honey or lemon for flavor.

Precautions and Considerations

While turmeric is generally safe for most people when consumed in moderate amounts, it can cause gastrointestinal issues in some individuals. Turmeric may also interact with certain medications, such as blood thinners, so it is important to consult with your healthcare provider before using turmeric supplements.

Turmeric is a versatile spice with powerful medicinal properties, including its potential to lower cholesterol levels. By incorporating turmeric into your diet in various ways, you can enjoy its health benefits and take proactive steps towards managing and lowering your cholesterol levels. In the following chapters, we will explore other natural remedies, including lime, lemon, garlic, onion, and clove, and how they can help you improve your cholesterol levels and overall health.

Chapter 9

Clove as a Natural Remedy for Cholesterol

Clove is a spice that is widely used in cooking and traditional medicine. It is known for its strong aroma and flavor, as well as its potential health benefits. In this chapter, we will explore the health benefits of clove, its impact on cholesterol levels, and practical tips for incorporating clove into your diet.

Health Benefits of Clove

Clove is rich in antioxidants and has anti-inflammatory, antimicrobial, and antifungal properties. It contains compounds such as eugenol, which has been studied for its potential to lower cholesterol levels and improve heart health. Clove also has a long history of use in traditional medicine for its digestive and pain-relieving properties.

Clove's Impact on Cholesterol Levels

Studies suggest that clove may help lower LDL cholesterol levels and triglycerides, while increasing HDL cholesterol levels. Clove contains compounds that inhibit the enzyme HMG-CoA reductase, which is involved in cholesterol synthesis in the liver. By blocking this enzyme, clove helps reduce the production of cholesterol in the body, leading to lower overall cholesterol levels.

Recipes and Usage Tips for Clove

- Whole Cloves: Whole cloves can be added to soups, stews, and rice dishes for a warm, aromatic flavor.
- Ground Cloves: Ground cloves can be used in baking, added to spice rubs for meats, or sprinkled on oatmeal or yogurt.

- Clove Tea: Clove tea can be made by steeping whole cloves in hot water for a few minutes. Add honey or lemon for flavor.

Precautions and Considerations

While clove is generally safe for most people when consumed in moderate amounts, it can cause allergic reactions in some individuals. Clove oil should be used with caution, as it can be irritating to the skin and mucous membranes. If you are pregnant, nursing, or taking medications, consult with your healthcare provider before using clove supplements.

Clove is a versatile spice with potential health benefits, including its ability to lower cholesterol levels. By incorporating clove into your diet in various ways, you can enjoy its health benefits and take proactive steps towards managing and lowering your cholesterol levels. In the following chapters, we will explore other natural remedies, including lime, lemon, garlic, onion, and turmeric, and how they can help you improve your cholesterol levels and overall health.

Chapter 10

Lime for Managing Cholesterol

Lime is a citrus fruit known for its refreshing flavor and high vitamin C content. It also offers several health benefits, including its potential to help manage cholesterol levels. In this chapter, we will explore the nutritional profile of lime, its impact on cholesterol levels, and practical tips for incorporating lime into your diet.

Nutritional Profile of Lime

Lime is low in calories but rich in vitamin C, antioxidants, and other nutrients. It also contains flavonoids, which have been studied for their potential to lower cholesterol levels and improve heart health. Lime juice is a popular ingredient in many cuisines and beverages, adding a bright, tangy flavor to dishes.

How Lime Helps Lower Cholesterol

Lime contains compounds such as flavonoids and limonoids, which have been shown to lower LDL cholesterol levels and triglycerides, while increasing HDL cholesterol levels. These compounds work by inhibiting the production of cholesterol in the liver and increasing the breakdown and excretion of cholesterol from the body.

Recipes and Usage Tips for Lime

- Lime Juice: Fresh lime juice can be added to water, tea, or cocktails for a refreshing drink.
- Lime Zest: The zest of lime can be used to add flavor to dishes, sauces, and marinades.
- Lime Wedges: Lime wedges can be used as a garnish for seafood, salads, or grilled meats.

Precautions and Considerations

While lime is generally safe for most people when consumed in moderate amounts, it can cause skin irritation or sun sensitivity in some individuals. If you are allergic to citrus fruits, consult with your healthcare provider before consuming lime or using lime supplements.

Lime is a versatile fruit with potential health benefits, including its ability to help manage cholesterol levels. By incorporating lime into your diet in various ways, you can enjoy its health benefits and take proactive steps towards managing and lowering your cholesterol levels. In the following chapters, we will explore other natural remedies, including lemon, garlic, onion, turmeric, and clove, and how they can help you improve your cholesterol levels and overall health.

Chapter 11

Lemon for Cholesterol Control

Lemon, another citrus fruit rich in vitamin C and antioxidants, offers several health benefits, including its potential to help control cholesterol levels. In this chapter, we will explore the nutritional profile of lemon, its impact on cholesterol levels, and practical tips for incorporating lemon into your diet.

Nutritional Benefits of Lemon

Lemon is low in calories but high in vitamin C and antioxidants, which help protect the body against free radical damage. It also contains flavonoids, which have been studied for their potential to lower cholesterol levels and improve heart health. Lemon juice is a popular ingredient in many dishes and beverages, adding a tangy flavor and refreshing aroma.

How Lemon Helps Lower Cholesterol

Lemon contains compounds such as flavonoids and limonoids, which have been shown to lower LDL cholesterol levels and triglycerides, while increasing HDL cholesterol levels. These compounds work by inhibiting the production of cholesterol in the liver and increasing the breakdown and excretion of cholesterol from the body.

Recipes and Usage Tips for Lemon

- Lemon Water: Drinking warm lemon water in the morning is a popular practice that is believed to aid digestion and promote detoxification.
- Lemon Zest: The zest of lemon can be used to add flavor to dishes, salads, dressings, and desserts.
- Lemon Juice: Fresh lemon juice can be used as a marinade for meats, a dressing for salads, or a flavoring for beverages and desserts.

Precautions and Considerations

While lemon is generally safe for most people when consumed in moderate amounts, it can cause tooth erosion or stomach irritation in some individuals. If you have a history of kidney stones or citrus allergies, consult with your healthcare provider before consuming lemon or using lemon supplements.

Lemon is a versatile fruit with potential health benefits, including its ability to help control cholesterol levels. By incorporating lemon into your diet in various ways, you can enjoy its health benefits and take proactive steps towards managing and lowering your cholesterol levels. In the following chapters, we will explore other natural remedies, including garlic, onion, turmeric, lime, and clove, and how they can help you improve your cholesterol levels and overall health.

Chapter 12

Natural Remedy for Cholesterol Management

Managing cholesterol levels through natural remedies can be an effective approach, especially when combined with a healthy lifestyle. This detailed guide provides specific instructions for overweight individuals and slim individuals, outlining the ingredients, preparation process, and usage recommendations.

For Overweight Individuals

Ingredients:

- 4 pieces of big garlic
- 1 large onion
- 1/2 teaspoon of clove
- 2 finger-sized turmeric roots
- 2 limes

Preparation Process:

1. Peel and Cut Garlic: Start by peeling the garlic and cutting them into smaller pieces. Garlic is known for its ability to lower cholesterol levels due to its high allicin content, which helps reduce LDL cholesterol.
2. Slice the Onion: Peel and slice the onion into small pieces. Onions contain flavonoids and sulfur compounds that can help lower cholesterol and improve heart health.
3. Turmeric: Peel the turmeric roots and cut them into smaller pieces. Turmeric is rich in curcumin, which has anti-inflammatory and cholesterol-lowering properties
4. Clove:Half teaspoon of clove.
5. Prepare the Lime: Cut each of the two limes into eight pieces. Limes are rich in vitamin C and antioxidants that support cardiovascular health.
6. Combine Ingredients: Place the garlic, onion, turmeric, lime pieces, and 1/2 teaspoon of clove into a small pot. Clove contains eugenol, which has been shown to reduce LDL cholesterol and triglycerides.
7. Add Water and Boil: Add half a liter of water to the pot. Bring the mixture to a boil and let

it simmer for ten minutes. Boiling helps to extract the beneficial compounds from the ingredients.

Usage Instructions:

- Dosage: Drink one cup of this concoction before your meal in the morning.
- Frequency: Repeat this process three times a week.
- Duration: Continue this regimen for two to four weeks, depending on your cholesterol levels. Monitor your progress, and once you feel a noticeable relief, you can stop the treatment.

For Slim Individuals

Ingredients:

- 4 pieces of big garlic
- 1 large onion
- 1/2 teaspoon of clove
- 2 finger-sized turmeric roots
- 1 large lemon (or 2 small lemons)

Preparation Process:

1. Peel and Cut Garlic: Peel the garlic and cut them into smaller pieces.
2. Slice the Onion: Peel and slice the onion into small pieces.
3. Turmeric: Peel the turmeric roots and cut them into smaller pieces.
4. Prepare the Lemon: Cut the lemon into eight pieces. Lemons are similar to limes in their high vitamin C content but may be preferable for individuals with different dietary needs or preferences
5. Clove: half teaspoon of clove.
6. Combine Ingredients: Place the garlic, onion, turmeric, lemon pieces, and 1/2 teaspoon of clove into a small pot.

7. Add Water and Boil: Add half a liter of water to the pot. Bring the mixture to a boil and let it simmer for ten minutes.

Usage Instructions:

- Dosage: Drink one cup of this mixture before your meal in the morning.
- Frequency: Repeat this process three times a week.
- Duration: Follow this regimen for two to four weeks. Assess your cholesterol levels and overall well-being, and discontinue the remedy once you achieve the desired results.

Additional Tips for Cholesterol Management

- **Diet:** Complement these natural remedies with a diet rich in fruits, vegetables, whole grains, and lean proteins. Avoid trans fats, reduce saturated fats, and incorporate healthy fats like those found in nuts, seeds, and fish.
- **Exercise:** Engage in regular physical activity such as brisk walking, jogging, swimming, or cycling. Aim for at least 150 minutes of moderate-intensity exercise per week.

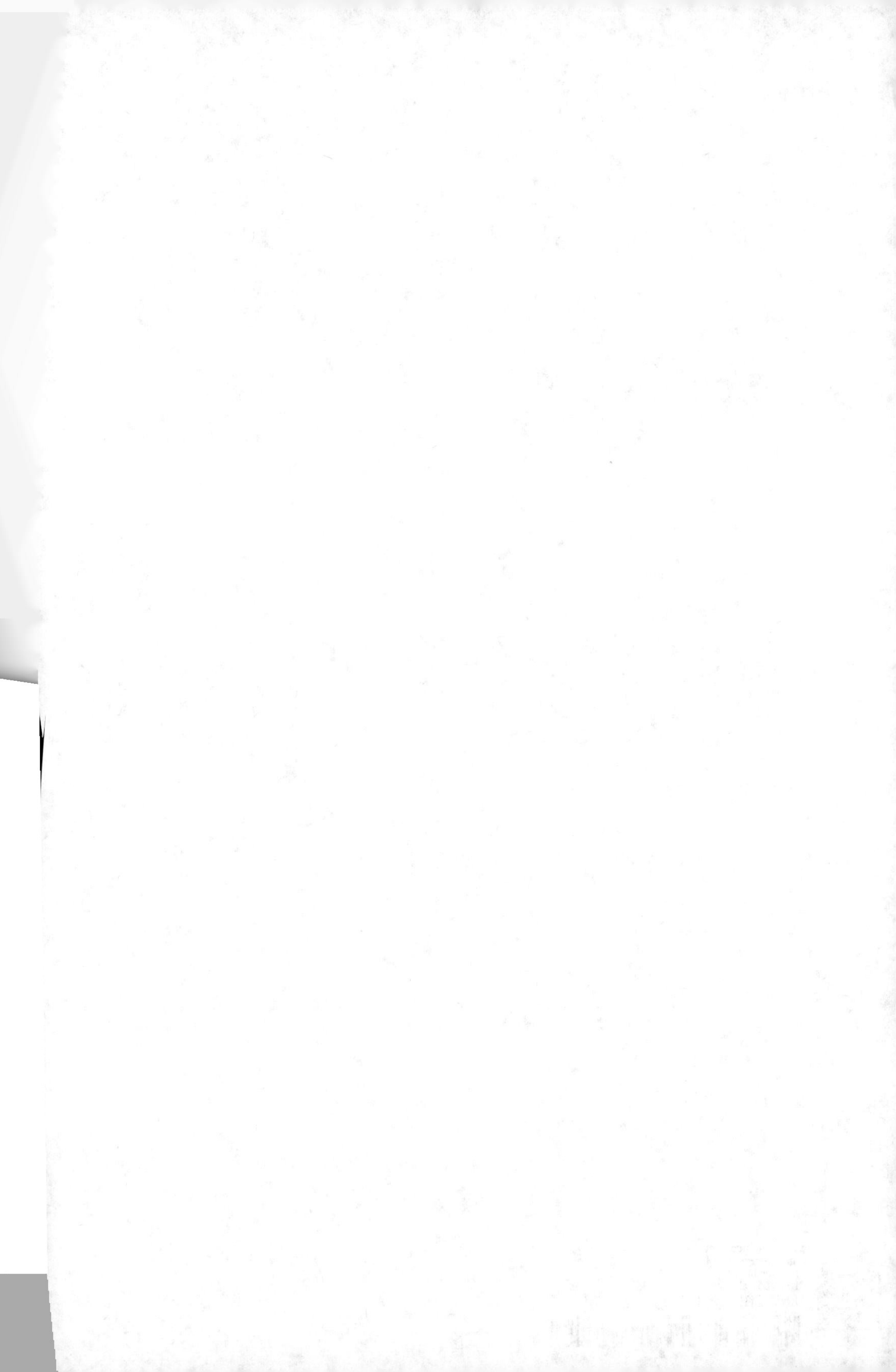